Lose Weight

Simple Exercises And Recipes To Lose Weight Quickly

Introduction

I want to thank you and congratulate you for downloading the book, "*Lose Weight: Simple Exercises and Recipes to Lose Weight Quickly*".

This book has lots of actionable information on simple exercises and recipes that will set you up on a path to losing weight effortlessly.

Over the years, many fad diets, weight loss programs, fancy exercise gadgets and equipment have been created to enable individuals to lose weight. Unfortunately, most of these achieve only temporary results because they neglect to hammer in the simple truth that losing or gaining weight boils down to the calories you consume and the activities you engage in.

Let's put it this way. At the end of the day, three things can occur when you calculate the amount of calories you've eaten and the activities you did throughout the day. These are:

- Weight gain - this occurs when you consume more calories than you burn. As a result, your body converts the excess glucose into fat and stores it in your cells and you end up gaining weight as a result.

- Weight maintenance - this occurs when the activities you do require the same amount of calories you consumed. There are no excess calories to be stored and there is no deficit. Thus, your weight remains the same.

- Weight loss - this is what happens when the activities you engage in burn more calories than what you consumed. Since there is a caloric deficit, you end up losing weight.

As you can see from above, in order for you to successfully lose weight, you need to reduce the amount of calories you consume and increase the amount of activities you engage in. I know this sounds cliché. But when you think about it; it sums up every weight loss program out there. This book has provides the easiest formula to attaining just that. You will learn how to work out effectively to turbocharge your metabolism to create the needed calorie deficit to lose weight. To support you in your workouts and journey to losing weight, the book will discuss some delicious recipes that will get you started in the journey to losing weight and keeping it off.

Thanks again for downloading this book. I hope you enjoy it!

Table of Contents

I know you know why you want to lose weight; that's why you are reading this book anyway! Therefore, we will start right away by discussing the types of exercises that you ought to engage in to turbocharge your metabolism to help you lose weight effortlessly.

Workouts Guaranteed To Make Weight Loss Easy

Physical activity is a very important part of the weight loss equation given that it helps increase the body's energy demands, which in turn creates an opportunity for the body to burn more calories. As a result, you end up losing weight (or more weight) if you create a calorie deficit in the process of exercising. Well, while all physical activities are important in weight loss, some exercises are better than others. If you want quick results, you need to choose exercises that create the most energy demands for the body during and after workout. So what exercises are these? Let's discuss some of these:

Cardio Exercises Guaranteed To Make Weight Loss Effortless

Cardio exercises refer to those exercises that get your heart pumping faster. They are great at burning calories, improving your wellbeing and keeping you fit. Here are a few cardio exercises that will get you to lose weight effortlessly:

Walking For Weight Loss

When you are not used to exercise, it helps to begin with activities that are familiar to you. One such activity is walking especially because walking is something billions of people do each day. Unfortunately, they don't do it enough to reap health benefits. If you want to lose weight through walking, you have to increase the amount of steps you take each day. Ideally, you should aim for 5000-10000 steps a day. So are these 'best practices' for walking? Well, there are; here are some of them:

1: Get into the right posture

When walking, you should not bend forwards as this will only hurt your lower back. Instead, stand tall, look straight ahead, keep your shoulders and hands relaxed and cup your hands gently at your sides. As you walk, swing your arms towards your breastbone and then do a downswing so that your hands brush your hips. Also, ensure that you land with your heel fast and that when you push off, you do so from your toes as well as from the ball of your foot.

2: Increase your steps gradually

Make no mistake. Walking exercises your muscles and as such, it would be foolhardy to overexert yourself in a bid to lose weight faster. You need to build up your steps. If you were walking for 10 minutes, add 2 more minutes to your walk. Once you are comfortable with that, add another 2-3 minutes and so forth until you are able to walk comfortably for 30-45 minutes.

If you wish to count steps instead of minutes, the same principle applies; increase the steps gradually. If you were walking 1000 steps, add 100 -200 steps, get comfortable with that and then add some more steps until the time you will be able to walk 5000 steps comfortably.

3: Use intervals to increase your pace

Once you've achieved your goal, you need to take the next step. This involves increasing the pace at which you walk. If you were timing your walks, you will need to increase the distance you walk without adding on any time. This will translate to you walking faster to cover the distance within the given time. If you were counting steps, you need to note how much it takes you to cover the steps and endeavour to reduce that time. Set a goal and walk towards it.

A good trick when you want to increase your pace is to do it in intervals. Walk comfortably for 3 minutes and then walk quickly for 2 minutes and so forth. This way, you will be able to gradually increase your pace until you become comfortable with walking at a faster pace the whole distance.

4: Create opportunities to walk

You need to create opportunities to walk each day. Use lunch breaks and 5-minute work breaks to walk. Limit your use of the elevator and use the stairs whenever possible. You can always get off several floors before your destination and walk the rest of the way. You can also include hills in your walks. When you walk uphill, you will burn more calories as you will be using more effort.

Jumping Rope For Weight Loss

A great way to burn calories is to jump rope. As a beginner, you can burn 12.5 calories per minute just from jumping rope i.e. 125 calories in 10 minutes; this is the amount of calories you would burn from 30 minutes of jogging. Amazing indeed! So how can you get the most from jumping rope? Well, the first thing you need to do is get the jumping technique right.

- Place your hands waist high with your elbows near your ribs. You need to hold the rope firmly but gently.

- Keep your jumps 1-2 inches from the ground.

- Rotate your wrists when turning the rope instead of rotating your shoulders and ensure that you turn the rope first before moving your feet.

Next, you need to determine your jump rope workout; there are two workouts that are quite effective i.e.

1. The timed jumping rope: This is where you try to do as many jumps in the span of 30 seconds. Set your goal for 50jumps and work towards it. Once you reach your goal, aim for 100 jumps.

2. Another workout you can use is the sliding scale jumping rope. This is where you start with let's say 250 jumps, then rest for 30-90 seconds (just until you catch your breath), then do 200, 150, 100 and eventually 50 jumps resting between each rep. This way, you will be able to do more jumps as the goal is reachable each time.

Stair Workout For Weight Loss

Another great way to burn calories is to do a stair workout. This is where you climb up and down the stairs to get your heart pumping faster and get to work out your quadriceps, glutes and hamstrings.
The one thing you will need is a staircase with at least 15 steps. Your workout consists of varied pacing. Start with a slower walk before climbing down again and then engage in a faster paced walk or run if you are fit enough for it. You can do the workout for 10minutes going up and down.

As time goes by, increase the amount of reps i.e. the number of times you walk up and down the stairs during your allocated time. As time goes by, you can increase the stair workout time.

As you climb the stairs, lean forward only slightly and do not place your weight on bar. Instead, just lightly rest your hand on the bar to keep your balance especially if you are not used to taking the stairs. Also, remember that you can spice up your workout. You can walk sideways, up and down the stairs before changing sides such that each leg gets an extensive workout each time.

Jumping Jacks For Weight Loss

Jumping jacks are not just for school going kids' gym class. They can also be great exercise for adults. In fact, an individual weighing 200 pounds can lose about 730 calories when performing jumping jacks for one hour. In order to perform jumping jacks, you should:

Step 1: Stand upright and place your arms at your sides.

Step 2: Jump up with your legs apart such that they are wider than your hip width. As you jump, raise your arms to shoulder level, straight out. It should look like you are forming a star shape with your legs and arms.

Step 3: Jump in to the starting position with your legs together and your arms at your sides.

As with all exercises, start small and gradually increase the time and the jumps you do. As you start out, depending on your fitness level, you may find it difficult to jump high of the ground. Don't let this discourage you; start low to the ground and gradually start jumping higher as you get more comfortable.

The important thing to keep in mind is that you need to pace yourself when you start doing cardio exercises. Set a goal, gradually work towards it and once you've achieved your goal, increase your pace before setting another goal. This way, you will burn fat and achieve your weight loss goals. Also keep in mind that you don't have to stick to doing one exercise. You can also incorporate other exercises like bodyweight exercises to keep your workout more interesting. Let's discuss some of these:

Body Weight Exercises For Weight Loss

The key to losing weight is to burn fat and you can do this by engaging in some fat burning exercises. You can do exercises such as:

Squats For Weight Loss

Squats are great for toning your legs and backside and they can be done almost anywhere. In order to do squats, you should:

Step 1: Stand upright with your legs shoulder width apart.

Step 2: Sit back as if you are sitting on a chair with your hands straight in front of you but ensure that your knees do not bend beyond your toe tips. Your upper body should bend forwards slightly. If you are uncomfortable when you put your hands straight, you can bend your elbows and clasp your fingers together at your chest to keep balance.

Step 3: Lower your body going as far back as possible by pushing your hips back. You should feel a burn as you do this.

Step 4: Go back to the staring position. Do 3 sets with 10 squats per set. As you grow more comfortable, increase the squats to 12 and then 25 per set.

As great as squats are for you, you may find it difficult to do them at first. If this is the case, you can use a chair to start off. Sit on a chair with your legs shoulder width apart and then stand up so that you are no longer sitting down. Hold the position for a few seconds and then sit back down. Complete a set and as you get more comfortable, ditch the chair.

Lunges For Weight Loss

Lunges give your glutes, quads, core muscles, calves, hamstrings a good workout. They also improve balance and coordination. In order to perform lunges, you should:
Step 1: Stand upright on even ground with your legs shoulder width apart and your hands on your hips. You should face forwards and keep your shoulders as relaxed as possible.
Step 2: Place one leg forward. Make the step as large as you comfortably can and bend both your knees to form 90 degrees angles. As you bend your knees, ensure that your front knee does not extend to pass your toes. You should also ensure that your back knee does not reach the ground even as it makes the 90 degree angle. Keep your back straight as you do the lunges.
Step 3: Hold the position for 5 seconds before returning to the starting point and changing legs.
You can start by doing 10 lunges per leg and then increase the sets, as you grow more comfortable. However, keep in mind that if you are not feeling any burn, you need to up your workout, as you may not be getting enough exercise.

Besides the exercises that you ought to engage in, it is also important to watch your diet. In the next chapter, we will discuss some powerful diet tips that will enhance your weight loss efforts.

Optimizing Your Diet For Weight Loss: Tips For Success

When you increase physical activity, you will indeed burn a considerable amount of calories. However, if you really want to lose weight, you must combine exercise with diet. In other words, the physical activity that you engage in should go towards getting rid of the 'old' extra fat. It should not go towards reducing 'new' fat. In other words, if you start watching your diet, you will ensure that your body has an easier time when it comes to losing weight. So how exactly can you execute this? We will learn that in detail:

1: Write down what you eat

The saying "words have power" rings true when it comes to losing weight. If you want to lose weight, you need to be conscious of what you are putting into your body. You can do this very well by writing down what you eat. When you note down what you eat, you begin to see your eating habits i.e. what you need to eat more of or less of and what you need to remove from your diet.

Another thing that you can do as you write down the food you eat is note down your moods. This will help you see how your moods affect your eating habits. Some people who have problem losing weight also report to be 'mood eaters'. If you discover this is a problem, you can look for other healthier ways to deal with your moods instead of indulging in food.

2: Do a carbohydrate sweep

One effective way to lose weight is to get rid of the foods that contribute to weight gain. As you know, if you eat excess carbs, they will be converted to fat and add to your weight gain. Thus, you should make it a point to take inventory of what you have in your home. Add more fruits and vegetables to your food stock and stop stocking junk foods and foods high in carbs. This way, if you are hungry, you will end up eating healthy snacks instead of snacking on junk food.

3: Exercise portion control

It's not just about what you eat but how much you eat. There are more calories in two servings than there are in one serving. You have to exercise portion control in order to lose weight. Serve your food on a plate (don't eat from the packet) and ensure that the plate is not a large plate and that you don't heap up your food. Small plates will create an illusion that you've served a lot of food even when you actually haven't, which means you are likely to feel satiated.

4: Use the power of smell

Smell is a powerful sense. At times, you can feel your mouth watering just because you've smelled your favourite dish. But the opposite is also true. Sometimes smelling a certain food or product can suppress your appetite. Bananas and apples are especially good at making you feel less hungry. Therefore, when you are hungry, smell a banana or smell an apple. Do so frequently to increase weight loss. You can also smell essential oils such as peppermint. Keep a bottle nearby and smell it whenever you feel hungry. This is especially useful if you suffer from food cravings. The smells will help you suppress the cravings.

5: Employ the 12-hour kitchen rule

Evening snacking plays a significant role in the number of calories you consume. This is because in the evening, most people just want to relax after they are done eating and others sleep just after eating. This means that the calories consumed do not have an outlet; they are not burned up and they end up adding on to weight gain. You can prevent this from happening by employing the 12-hour kitchen rule whereby you lock up the kitchen for 12 hours. This will reduce the chances of you giving in to a late night snack.

7: Drink water

When it comes to weight loss, water is your ally. As such, you should be determined to drink a lot of water. For instance, drink a glass before you eat your meal. This will serve to make you feel a bit fuller even before you start eating. Another thing to keep in mind is that a lot of times, thirst is disguised as hunger. Therefore, when you feel hunger pangs, don't be too quick to get a bite to eat. Instead, drink water and wait for a while to see how your body responds. Chances are that you will postpone your eating.

Note: Don't assume you will drink water if it is not there. As they say, "out of sight, out of mind". If you don't carry water with you when you travel or go to work, you will end up drinking less water at the end of the day. Therefore, always have a bottle of water with you as you go about your day and ensure that it is empty by the time you return home.

Other strategies that can help you to eat less food include the following:

✓ Serve food in blue plates, as the color 'blue' has a satiating effect on the brain.

✓ You also need to be careful when eating out especially in restaurants that tend to serve food in larger plates. Rest assured that if you reduce the amount of food you eat, you will lose weight.

✓ Add spice to your food (especially pepper) to create a satiating feeling.

4: Practice clean eating

Cleaning eating simply means leaning towards healthier options whenever you choose what to eat. In this case, you would want to stick to organic products as much as you can, avoid artificial sweeteners or products such as white sugar and white rice and that you read nutrition labels before purchasing any food product.

One trick to use is to check the number of ingredients a product has. The unwritten rule being that the more ingredients a product has, the more additives it is likely to have. Thus, stick to foods with fewer ingredients in them.

Following these diet tips will enable you to lose weight effortlessly. As you follow these tips, always keep in mind that it is the little changes you make that make it possible for you to achieve your bigger goals.

With what we've learnt in mind, let's now learn about some delicious recipes that will make your weight loss journey easier and filled with fun.

Breakfast Recipes

Broccoli And Feta Omelet With Toast
Nutritional Information: Calories 390, Fat 19g, Protein 23g, Fiber 6g
Servings: 1
Ingredients
2 slices rye bread, toasted
¼ teaspoon dried dill
2 tablespoons feta cheese, crumbled
2 large eggs, beaten
1 cup chopped broccoli
Cooking spray
Directions
Heat skillet over medium heat and coat it with cooking spray. Add the chopped broccoli and stir from time to time for 3 minutes.
Whisk the egg, dill and feta in a bowl and then pour it over the broccoli but do not disturb it. You can tilt the pan to spread the mixture. Cook for 3-4 minutes and then flip sides and cook for another 2 minutes or until the omelette is cooked through. Remove and serve with toast.

Grain Bowl
Nutritional Information: Calories 379, Fat 16g, Carbohydrates 54g, Fiber 9g, Protein 8g
Servings: 2
Ingredients
1 tomato, cubed
½ avocado, roughly chopped
2 cups leftover cooked grains (brown rice, quinoa, farro, couscous etc.)
Black pepper
Kosher salt
1 bunch spinach, roughly chopped
1 clove garlic, finely chopped
1 tablespoon olive oil plus more for drizzling
Directions
Heat oil in a skillet over medium heat and sauté the garlic for 1 minute before adding the spinach, salt and pepper and cooking for another 1-2minutes. Place the grains in bowls and top up with the cooked spinach, tomato and avocado.

Smoothie Bowls

Nutritional Information: Calories 209, Fat 1g, Protein 9g, Carbohydrates 46g, Fiber 8g

Servings: 2

Ingredients

Toasted coconut flakes, for serving

Granola, for serving

½ cup low fat milk

1 tablespoon chia seeds (optional)

½ cup nonfat Greek yogurt

2 bananas

2 cups frozen raspberries

Directions

Blend bananas, raspberries, yogurt, milk and chia seeds until smooth. Serve in bowls and top with granola and toasted coconut flakes.

Gingerbread Chia Pudding

Nutritional Information: Calories 307, Fat 17.8g, Carbohydrates 36.6g, Dietary Fiber 12.8g, Sugars 18.1g, Protein 13.5g

Servings: 1

Ingredients

Toppings:

1 tablespoon chopped pecans (or other nut)

1 tablespoon raisins

Pudding:

Sea salt to taste

Dash of ground clove

¼ teaspoon cinnamon

¼ teaspoon ground ginger

1 tablespoon maple syrup

¾ cup unsweetened soymilk (or milk of choice)

¼ cup chia seeds

Directions

Place the ingredients minus the toppings in a mason jar. Stir to mix them together and then refrigerate for 6 hours or overnight. Remove and add the toppings and serve for breakfast.

High Fiber Cereal

Nutritional Information: Calories 287, Protein 14.8g, Fat 3.3g, Carbohydrate 41.9g, Sugars 18.0g

Servings: 1

Ingredients

½ cup low fat milk

1/3 cup blueberries

6 raspberries

1/3 banana, sliced

1/3 cup All Bran

1 Weet Bix, crushed

Directions

Place the Weet Bix in a bowl and then add the All-Bran on top and the banana slices, the berries and finally the milk. Serve immediately.

Lunch Recipes

White Bean And Herb Hummus With Crudités
Nutritional Information: Calories 150, Fat 10g, Protein 4g,
Carbohydrates 14g, Fiber 3g
Servings: 1
Ingredients
Assorted raw vegetables (broccoli, tomatoes, cucumbers,
carrots, green pepper, red pepper etc.)
2 teaspoons olive oil
1 tablespoon lemon juice
1 tablespoon chopped chives
¼ cup canned white beans, rinsed and drained
Directions
In a bowl, mix together beans, chives, oil and lemon juice until
the mixture is smooth. Serve with assorted raw vegetables.

Veggie And Pesto Sandwich

Nutritional Information: Calories 260, Fat 5g, Carbohydrates 43g, Dietary Fiber 4g, Sugars 6g, Protein 13g

Servings: 4

Ingredients

¼ cup pesto

1 cup packed arugula

2 Roma tomatoes, thinly sliced

¼ cup low0fat shredded mozzarella cheese

8 pieces artisan whole grain bread

4 ¼ slices red bell peppers, cored, seeded, roasted

1 tablespoon plus 2 teaspoons extra virgin olive oil

8 ounces white mushrooms, sliced

Directions

Preheat the oven to 375 degrees.

Heat a tablespoon of oil in a skillet and sauté the mushrooms for 8 minutes or until they turn soft.

Toast bread on a cookie sheet. Remove it and place 1 tablespoon of cheese over it and toast until the cheese melts.

Remove the bread and top up with mushrooms, tomatoes, pesto, arugula and bell peppers and serve.

Garden Salad With Lemon And Oil Dressing

Nutritional Information: Calories 220, Fat 17.3g, Carbohydrates 16.3g, Dietary Fiber 7.5g, Protein 4.9g, Sugars 3.8g

Servings: 2

Ingredients

1 cup roasted chicken breast, chopped (optional)
1 tomato, diced
½ cup fresh parsley
1 cup bean sprouts
8 almonds, sliced
1 carrot, grated
½ cucumber, sliced
1/3 red onion, thinly sliced

Dressing:

Salt to taste
¼ teaspoon black pepper
1 teaspoon dried oregano
1 tablespoon extra-virgin olive oil
Juice of 1 lemon

Directions

Place the salad ingredients into a bowl and toss to mix them together. In another bowl, whisk the dressing ingredients and then drizzle them over the salad. Serve and enjoy.

Dinner Recipes

Easy Pork Chops With Sweet And Sour Glaze
Nutritional Information: Calories 392.6, Fat 18.5g,
Carbohydrates 16.2g, Protein 38.3g
Servings: 4
Ingredients
For the glaze:
Kosher salt and freshly ground pepper to taste
Pinch of crushed red pepper flakes (optional)
½ teaspoon dried thyme
½ teaspoon dried basil
½ teaspoon dried oregano
2 cloves garlic, minced
3 tablespoon honey
¼ cup balsamic vinegar
For the pork chops:
2 tablespoons unsalted butter
Kosher salt and freshly ground black pepper to taste
4 (8-ounce) bone in pork chops
Directions
Preheat oven to 400 degrees F.
Prepare pork chops by seasoning with salt and pepper. Heat a
large skillet, melt the butter and then brown the pork chops on
both sides for 2-3 minutes. Once they are browned, place in
the oven and cook for 8-10 minutes according to their
thickness.
In a small saucepan, prepare the glaze by combining balsamic
vinegar, red pepper flakes, honey, basil, thyme, oregano,
garlic, salt and pepper and boiling them. You should reduce
the heat once it starts to boil and let the glaze simmer for 5
minutes.
Remove and serve the pork chops with the sweet and sour
glaze.

Butter Squash, Arugula And Goat Cheese Pasta
Nutritional Information: Calories 307, Fat 14.1g, Carbs 36.3g.
Fiber 5g,Sugar 3.4g, Protein 53.9g
Servings: 5
Ingredients
1/3 cup toasted pine nuts
2 big handfuls fresh baby arugula
2 ounces goat cheese
12 ounces whole wheat dried pasta
Salt and freshly ground pepper to taste
1 tablespoon vegetable oil
1 medium butternut squash, peeled, seeded and diced
Directions
Heat oven to 425 degrees F and spray baking sheet with
cooking spray (you can also use parchment paper).
In a bowl, mix together butternut squash and oil and toss to
coat the squash evenly and then proceed to evenly spread the
squash on the prepared baking sheet. Bake for 20-25 minutes
ensuring that you flip the dish at the halfway point. Remove
and set aside.
Cook the pasta according to the instructions on the package.
Once it is cooked, set aside 1 cup of water and drain the rest.
In the pot, return the pasta, ¼ cup of pasta water and goat
cheese and toss to allow the cheese to melt. You can add
tablespoons of more water if you wish to lighten the sauce.
Combine arugula, butternut squash and pine nuts and serve
immediately.

5 Ingredient Chili
Nutritional Information: Calories 249, Fat 5.3g, Carbs 23g, Fiber 9g, Sugar 11g, Protein 29.4g

Servings: 4-6

Ingredients

Optional toppings – green onions, cheese, cilantro, sour cream
2 tablespoon chilli powder
12 (15-ounce) cans beans of choice, drained
3 (15-ounce) cans diced tomatoes with green chiles
1 small white onion, diced
1 lb ground beef or turkey

Directions

In a stockpot, brown the ground beef over medium-heat. Stir frequently and then transfer it to a plate. You should reserve at least 1 tablespoon of grease before discarding the rest. Use it to cook the onion for 4-5 minutes or until it is translucent. Once the onion is ready, add the rest of the ingredients plus the cooked beef and stir. Bring the mixture to a boil and then simmer for 10 minutes over medium-low heat.

Remove and serve. You can garnish with toppings of your choice if you so wish.

Wild Mushroom And Barley Risotto

Nutritional Information: Calories 309, Fat 9g, Carbohydrates 47g, Fiber 10g, Protein 9g

Servings: 3

Ingredients

Freshly ground pepper, to taste

2 teaspoons balsamic vinegar

1 tablespoon butter

1/3 cup freshly grated Parmesan cheese

6 cups baby arugula

½ cup red wine

11/2 cups pearl barley, rinsed

3 cups mixed wild mushrooms, coarsely chopped

2 cloves garlic, minced

1 small onion, minced

2 tablespoons extra-virgin olive oil

11/2 cups water

6 cups vegetable, mushroom or chicken-broth (with reduced-sodium)

Directions

Simmer broth and water in a saucepan.

Heat oil in Dutch oven then add onion and garlic and stir from time to time for 2 minutes before adding the mushrooms for 2-3 more minutes. Stir and add barley, cook for 1 more minute and then add wine for another minute and then reduce heat to medium.

Add ½ cup of hot broth and stir so that it is absorbed and then add another ½ cup and continue adding broth in half cups and then let it simmer for 35-45 minutes before stirring in the arugula and cooking for 1 more minute. Remove and stir in butter, vinegar, cheese, salt and pepper and serve.

Snacks Recipes

Kale chips
Nutritional Information: Calories 51, Carbohydrates 4g, Fat 4g, Fiber 1g
Servings: 4
Ingredients
½ teaspoon salt
1 tablespoon olive oil
1 bunch kale, washed and cut into 2-inch pieces (remove ribs)
Directions
Preheat oven to 325 degrees F then place the kale on a baking sheet and bake for 10-15 minutes. Ensure you mix the kale at the halfway mark. Remove when crispy not browned.

Raspberry-Apple Smoothie

Nutritional Information: Calories 191, Proteins 3g, Carbs 46g, Fat 3g, Fiber 16g

Servings: 1

Ingredients

4 ice cubes

2 teaspoon ground psyllium powder

1 tablespoon unsweetened soy protein powder (optional)

¾ cup unsweetened almond milk or fat-free plain yogurt

½ apple, cored and coarsely chopped

½ cup frozen or fresh raspberries

Directions

Combine all ingredients in a blender and blend until smooth. Serve.

Gluten Free Chocolate And Pear Muffins

Nutritional Information: Calories 186, Protein 11.6g, Fat 5.6g. Carbohydrate 26.8g, Sugars 15.2g

Servings: 8

Ingredients

½ pear, sliced thinly

1 teaspoon bicarbonate soda

1 teaspoon baking powder

½ cup yogurt

4 tablespoon Light Marg Spread (or butter)

½ cup almond milk

2 egg whites

½ cup sugar

¼ cup cocoa powder

½ cup rice flour

½ cup almond meal

Directions

Preheat oven to 180 degrees C.

Sift rice flour, almond meal and cocoa powder and then add sugar and mix well. Microwave ½ cup of almond milk for 1 minute and set aside. Melt butter and set aside and whisk the egg whites. Mix the ingredients except the egg whites and then slowly fold the egg white into the mixture but don't beat it.

Pour the ingredients into patty pans and then put 2 pear slices at the center vertical near the end parts and bake for 25 minutes. Remove when it's cooked.

Granola Bars
Nutritional Information: calories 162, fat 6g
Servings: 10
Ingredients
1/8 teaspoon salt
½ teaspoon vanilla extract
¼ cup honey
¼ cup turbinado sugar (or brown sugar)
¼ cup creamy almond butter
2 tablespoons dried blueberries
2 tablespoons raisins
¼ cup dried cherries
1 cup unsweetened whole-grain puffed cereal
2 tablespoons wheat germ
1 tablespoon flaxseeds
¼ cup walnuts, coarsely chopped
1 cup old-fashioned rolled oats
Directions
Grease pan with cooking spray. In a bowl, mix together cereal, oats, walnuts, wheat germ, flaxseeds and dried fruit.
In another bowl, mix together sugar, honey, almond butter, salt and vanilla and heat over a saucepan for 2-5 minutes and then pour the mixture over the almond mixture and mix using a spoon. Press the prepared mixture into the pan and place in the refrigerator for half an hour before cutting into pieces.

Loaded Spaghetti
Nutritional Information: calories 420
Servings: 1
Ingredients
2/3 cup cooked endamame
1 cup cooked whole-wheat spaghetti
1 teaspoon olive oil
½ cup sliced red onion
1 cup sliced bell pepper
Directions
Heat skillet and sauté onions and peppers in the oil until onions appear translucent. Mix the ingredients with pasta and edamame and serve.

Conclusion

The important thing to remember is that you need to create a caloric deficit in order to lose weight. This means that the calories you consume should be less than the calories you end up using. This is where watching what you eat and ensuring to engage in physical activity greatly contributes positively in your weight loss journey.

Thank you again for downloading this book!
I hope this book was able to help you to understand how to lose weight.
The next step is to implement what you have learned.

Finally, if you enjoyed this book, would you be kind enough to leave a review for this book on Amazon?

Click here to leave a review for this book on Amazon!

Thank you and good luck!

www.ingramcontent.com/pod-product-compliance
Lightning Source LLC
Chambersburg PA
CBHW071319280526
45788CB00004B/1944